How to Make

Natural Bath Teas

Dr Miriam Kinai

Contents

1

Bath Teas Making Equipment

Glass bowl

Wooden spoon

Dark glass jar

Cotton bath tea bag or organza bags or muslin bags or cheese cloth

Scoops are optional

* * * * *

2

Basic Bath Teas Recipe Ingredients

A basic body tea basically consists of the following ingredients:

2 cups of Herbs - to provide the healing benefits. Perfect examples include Peppermint leaves, Calendula flowers, Chamomile flowers, Lavender flowers, Rose petals, Rosemary leaves.

10 - 20 drops of Essential Oils - to add healing aromas and therapeutic benefits. Grated lemon and orange rind can also be used.

Additional but optional ingredients for advanced bath teas include:

Sea salt which has a high mineral content and a detoxifying effect on the body. 1 cup of sea salt can be added for every 2 cups of herbs.

Epsom salts for their relaxing properties. 1 cup can be added for every 2 cups of herbs.

Powdered milk which hydrates and softens the skin as the lactic acid exfoliates or gets rid of the dead surface skin cells to reveal more youthful skin. 1 cup of powdered milk can be added for every 2 cups of herbs.

Green tea is a potent antioxidant which can be combined with the dry herbs to make part of the 2 cups of herbs.

Black tea soothes the skin and it is very effective in healing skin damage from sun burn. It can also be combined with the dry herbs to make part of the 2 cups of herbs.

* * * * *

3

Basic Bath Teas Recipe Instructions

1. Add the essential oils drop by drop to the 2 cups of herbs until you get your desired scent.

2. Add the optional ingredients if using e.g. 1 cup sea salt, 1 cup Epsom salts, 1 cup powdered milk.

3. Add more essential oils drop by drop as you mix

4. Put the mixture in an air tight jar or you can add a scoopful of the mixture into a cotton bath tea bag and store the filled bath tea bags in the air tight jar.

* * * * *

4

Therapeutic Bath Teas Recipes

Arthritis Bath Tea Recipe

2 cups of Herbs used to manage arthritis such as arnica flowers, lavender flowers, and rosemary leaves.

10 - 20 drops of Essential Oils used for arthritis treatment like Lemon, Eucalyptus, Lavender, Peppermint, Roman chamomile, and Rosemary.

Follow the above Basic Bath Tea Recipe Instructions.

***

Eczema Bath Tea Recipe

2 cups of Herbs used to manage eczema such as calendula flowers, chamomile flowers, and St John's wort leaves and flowers.

10 - 20 drops of Essential Oils used for eczema treatment like Geranium, Lavender, Roman chamomile, and Rosemary essential oils.

Follow the above Basic Bath Tea Recipe Instructions.

Psoriasis Bath Tea Recipe

2 cups of Herbs used to manage psoriasis such as chamomile flowers, and lavender flowers.

10 - 20 drops of Essential Oils used for the management of psoriasis such as Roman chamomile, Tea tree, and Lavender essential oils.

Follow the above Basic Bath Tea Recipe Instructions.

***

Dry Skin Bath Tea Recipe

2 cups of Herbs used to manage dry skin such as calendula flowers, chamomile flowers, and lavender flowers.

10 - 20 drops of Essential Oils used to manage dry skin such as Lavender, Roman chamomile, and Ylang ylang essential oils.

Follow the above Basic Bath Tea Recipe Instructions.

***

Mature Skin Bath Tea Recipe

2 cups of Herbs such as calendula flowers, chamomile flowers, and lavender flowers.

10 - 20 drops of Geranium essential oil.

Follow the above Basic Bath Tea Recipe Instructions.

***

Menopausal Symptoms Bath Tea Recipe

2 cups of Herbs used for menopausal symptoms such as chamomile flowers and rosemary leaves.

10 - 20 drops of Essential Oils used to manage menopausal symptoms such as Clary sage, Geranium, Lavender, Peppermint, Roman chamomile, and Rosemary essential oils.

Follow the above Basic Bath Tea Recipe Instructions.

***

Pre-Menstrual Tension (PMS) and Painful Periods Bath Tea Recipe

2 cups of Herbs used to manage eczema such as as lavender flowers and chamomile flowers.

10 - 20 drops of Essential Oils used to manage menstrual symptoms such as Clary sage, Geranium, Lavender, and Roman chamomile essential oils.

Follow the above Basic Bath Tea Recipe Instructions.

***

Stress Management Bath Tea Recipe

2 cups of Herbs used for managing stress such as lavender flowers and chamomile flowers.

10 - 20 drops of Essential Oils used for managing stress such as Lavender, Roman Chamomile, Bergamot, Clary sage, Petitgrain, Geranium, Marjoram, Peppermint, Rose, Sandalwood, Ylang ylang essential oils.

Follow the above Basic Bath Tea Recipe Instructions.

***

Sadness Bath Tea Recipe

2 cups of Herbs used to manage depression such as rosemary leaves and St John's wort.

10 - 20 drops of Essential Oils used for the treatment of depression such as Bergamot, Clary sage, Roman chamomile, Lavender, Rosemary, Rose, Ylang ylang.

Follow the above Basic Bath Tea Recipe Instructions.

***

Mental Exhaustion Bath Tea Recipe

2 cups of Herbs used to improve mental concentration such as rosemary leaves.

10 - 20 drops of Essential Oils used to improve mental concentration such as Peppermint, Eucalyptus, Lemon and Rosemary essential oils.

Follow the above Basic Bath Tea Recipe Instructions.

***

Insomnia (Sleeplessness) Bath Tea Recipe

2 cups of Herbs such as lavender flowers.

10 - 20 drops of Essential Oils such as Lavender, Roman chamomile, and Ylang ylang essential oils.

Follow the above Basic Bath Tea Recipe Instructions.

* * * * *

5

Characteristics Of Essential Oils Used In Making Bath Teas

Choose the aromatherapy essential oils to use depending on the effects you want the bath salts to have. For example:

Clary Sage Essential Oil has an herbaceous scent. It can help relieve stress related tension, reduce irritability and help one relax. It is also used for the management of mature and acne prone skin. Do not use it during pregnancy or if you are drinking alcohol or driving or if you have endometriosis, ovarian cysts, uterine cysts, breast cancer or you are at high risk for developing breast cancer as it may have an "estrogen-like" effect on the body.

Eucalyptus essential oil has an invigorating scent. It can help relieve stress related mental tension and mental exhaustion. It is also used in the management of joint aches and pains. Do not use eucalyptus essential oil if you have epilepsy, high blood pressure or apply it near a baby's nostrils.

Geranium Essential Oil has a fresh, minty rose scent. It can help relieve nervous tension and anxiety. It is also used in the management of eczema, cellulite as well as mature skin. Avoid using it in pregnancy.

Grapefruit essential oil has a refreshing, bitter-sweet scent. It can help relieve tension and release repressed emotions. It is also used in the management of cellulite.

Lavender essential oil has a soothing, floral scent. It can help one relax and relieve stress related tension, sleeplessness, anxiety and depression. It is also used in the management of acne, eczema and dry skin conditions. Do not use lavender essential oil in pregnancy, if you are breastfeeding, on young children as it may cause breast development in young boys and girls. Avoid it if you have low blood pressure as you may feel drowsy after using it.

Lemon essential oil has an clarifying fresh scent. It can help relieve mental tension, alleviate mental fatigue and increase concentration. It is also used in the management of acne and post acne dark skin spots. Do not use it if skin will be exposed to sunlight or UV rays in the next 12-24 hours. Do not use it if you have low blood pressure or you are allergic to lemons.

Lemongrass essential oil has a vitalizing, lemony scent. It can help relieve tension and muscle aches. It is also used in the management of acne. Do not use it if skin will be exposed to sunlight or UV rays in the next 12-24 hours.

Roman chamomile essential oil has a sweet and fruity scent. It can help relieve stress related tension headaches. It is also used in the management of eczema, psoriasis and dry skin conditions. Avoid using it in pregnancy and if you are allergic to ragweed.

Spearmint essential oil has a gently-energizing minty scent. It can help relieve mental tension and exhaustion. It is also used in the management of nausea.

Rosemary Essential Oil has an uplifting and stimulating scent. It can help relieve mental exhaustion and feeling rundown. It is also used in the management of eczema, muscle aches and joint pains. Do not use rosemary essential oil if you are pregnant or have epilepsy or high blood pressure. Avoid using it if you have a fever or you want to sleep and in children under 5 years.

Sweet orange essential oil has a cheeringly, refreshing scent. It can help mange stress related tension. It is also used in the management of cellulite and common colds. Do not use it if skin will be exposed to sunlight or UV rays in the next 12-24 hours.

Peppermint essential oil has a head-clearing, refreshing scent. It can help relieve tension and fatigue. It is also used to manage flatulence. Do not use peppermint essential oil in pregnancy, if breastfeeding, on children less than 5 years, if you have epilepsy or irregular heart beats or cardiac fibrillation or high blood pressure and before using a sun bed or going to hot humid places.

Tea tree essential oil has a purifying almost medicinal scent. It can help relieve tension and fatigue. It is also been used in the management of acne and athlete's foot.

Ylang ylang Essential Oil has a fragrantly floral scent. It can help relieve anxiety, tension and help one relax. It is also used as an aphrodisiac and in the management of dry skin conditions. Do not use ylang ylang essential oil if you have low blood pressure or sensitive, damaged skin.

* * * * *

6

Characteristics Of Herbs Used In Making Bath Teas

Different herbs can be added to bath teas to increase their esthetic appeal and healing benefits. These herbal healing benefits that will be extracted are as follows:

Arnica flowers are believed to have anti-inflammatory properties and are used to relieve the pains of sprains, muscle aches and joint pains. Do not use arnica if you are allergic to it, if pregnant or breastfeeding.

Calendula flowers are believed to have antioxidant, anti-inflammatory and anti-infective properties. They are used to help wounds heal faster, for minor cuts, small insect bites, minor bruises, first degree burns, mild sunburns and mild skin infections. Calendula has been shown to prevent dermatitis or skin inflammation in breast cancer patients receiving radiation treatment. Do not use calendula if you are allergic to it, allergic to daisy or aster family plants such as ragweed and chrysanthemums, if pregnant or breastfeeding or trying to conceive.

Avoid calendula preparations if you are taking sedatives, high blood pressure and diabetes medications.

Chamomile flowers are believed to have relaxing and mild antiseptic properties. They are used to help relieve anxiety, relieve emotional stress, relax tense muscles and relieve muscle spasms. Do not use/avoid chamomile if you are allergic to it, allergic to daisy or aster family plants such as ragweed and chrysanthemums, have asthma, are pregnant as it may cause miscarriage, if driving as it may cause drowsiness, if taking alcohol, for at least 2 weeks before surgery or dental procedures as it may cause bleeding. Do not use/avoid chamomile if you are taking blood thinners such as warfarin (coumadin), clopidogrel (plavix) or aspirin as it may cause bleeding, sedatives, drugs used to treat sleeplessness, high blood pressure medications as it may lower the blood pressure and diabetes medications as it can lower the blood sugar.

Comfrey leaves are believed to have anti-inflammatory, skin regenerative and antiseptic properties. They are used to relieve muscle strains and ligament sprains. Do not use/ avoid comfrey if you are allergic to it, on broken skin, on children, the elderly, if pregnant or breastfeeding, in liver disease, alcoholism and cancer. Do not use/ avoid comfrey if you are taking acetaminophen (panadol, tylenol). Do not use/ avoid comfrey if using herbs known to cause liver problems such as kava, valerian and skullcap.

Lavender flowers are believed to have calming, analgesic, anti-inflammatory and skin regenerative properties. They are used to relieve tension, reduce anxiety, insomnia, manage eczema, muscle and joint aches. Do not use/ avoid lavender if you are allergic to it, on broken skin, if pregnant or breastfeeding, on young boys as it may cause male breast development. Do not use/ avoid lavender if you are taking sedatives, anti-anxiety medications such as lorazepam and narcotic analgesics such as morphine and oxycodone.

Rose petals are believed to have skin softening properties.

Rosemary leaves are believed to have antioxidant, mentally stimulating and antimicrobial properties. They are used to reduce feelings of sadness, increase mental concentration and relieve muscle pains and joint aches. Do not use/ avoid rosemary if you are allergic to it, are breastfeeding or pregnant as it may cause miscarriages, are under 18 years old, have high blood pressure, peptic ulcers, ulcerative colitis or Crohn's disease. Do not use/avoid rosemary if you are taking blood thinners such as warfarin (coumadin), clopidogrel (plavix) or aspirin as it may cause bleeding, angiotensin converting enzyme (ACE) inhibitors such as captopril and lisinopril for high blood pressure, diuretics such as furosemide (lasix) and hydrochlorothiazide also used for high blood pressure treatment and medicines for diabetes medications as it may alter the blood sugar levels and lithium.

St John's Wort flowers and leaves have anti-depressant, anti-inflammatory, antiseptic properties. They are used to relieve mild depression, and manage mild eczema. Do not use/ avoid St John's wort if you are allergic to it, have major or severe depression and bipolar disorder, are pregnant, breastfeeding or trying to get pregnant. Do not use/ avoid St John's wort if you are going to have surgery in five days, are taking digoxin for the heart, antiretroviral medicines used to treat HIV/ AIDS, if you are taking medications to treat depression as it could result in the dangerous serotonin syndrome. These antidepressant medications include serotonin reuptake inhibitors (SSRIs) such as citalopram, fluoxetine and sertraline, tricyclic antidepressants such as amitriptyline and imipramine, monoamine oxidase inhibitors (MAOIs) such as phenelzine and tranylcypromine.

* * * * *

About The Author

Dr. Miriam Kinai is a medical doctor and a certified aromatherapist.

You can visit her blog at
http://www.TheBestSellingEbooks.blogspot.com/

or follow her on twitter at http://twitter.com/AlmasiHealth

Email enquiries to drkinai@yahoo.com with BOOKS as your subject.

Other Books By Dr Miriam Kinai

Natural Body Products Series

Books in our Natural Body Product Series teach you how to make handmade bath and beauty products. They also teach you the benefits of various vegetable oils, essential oils, natural butters, and herbs to help you choose the best ingredients for your homemade products.

These books are filled with recipes for managing normal, sensitive, mature, and dry skin types as well as cellulite, eczema, psoriasis, ringworms, dandruff, thinning hair, menopause, pre-menstrual tension, painful periods, arthritis, stress, sadness, mental fatigue, and insomnia.

Books in the Natural Bath and Body Products Series include:

1. How to Make Handmade Natural Bath Bombs

2. How to Make Handmade Natural Bath Melts

3. How to Make Handmade Natural Bath Salts

4. How to Make Handmade Natural Bath Teas

5. How to Make Handmade Natural Body Butters

6. How to Make Handmade Natural Body Lotions

7. How to Make Handmade Natural Body Scrubs

8. How to Make Handmade Natural Healing Balms

9. How to Make Handmade Natural Herb Infused Oils

10. How to Make Handmade Natural Soap

* * * * *

Managing Stress with the Word of God

Managing Stress with the Word of God teaches you how to manage stress effectively by combining time tested Biblical principles with medical proven relaxation techniques.

Topics covered in this book include:

1. What is stress?

2. What is the body's response to stress?

3. Symptoms of Stress

4. Biblical Principles for Stress Management

5. Medical Relaxation Techniques

6. Other Stress Relief Activities

* * * * *

Rules Of Relaxation

Rules of Relaxation teaches you 130 simple relaxation techniques as it covers the A to Z of stress management from Assert yourself, Breathe deeply, Cast your burdens, Drink herbal teas, Establish social support, Formulate realistic goals, Guard your heart, Have complementary hobbies, Identify personal stressors, Jaunt, Keep the Sabbath, Listen to music, Meditate on the Word, Nab a nap, Optimize stress, Pamper yourself, Quash sin, Reason rationally, Schedule news fasts, Trust God, Use cognitive restructuring, Veto worry, Work out, eXperiment with aromatherapy, Yield to God to Zap job stress.

* * * * *

Sword Words

SWORD WORDS teaches you how to wage Christian spiritual warfare using the SWORD of the Spirit which is the WORD of God. (Ephesians 6:17)

It instructs you how to wield your SWORD WORDS together with the full armor of God. It demystifies the enemy's devices and explains the battle plan. It also tells you how to position yourself strategically and communicate effectively with your backup so that you can win your battles regardless of whether you are fighting for your marriage, children, or finances or fighting addictions, opposition, and fear.

* * * * *

Resolving Conflicts just like Jesus Christ

Resolving Conflicts just like Jesus Christ uses Biblical examples from Jesus Christ to King Solomon to teach Conflict Resolution Strategies, Third Party Mediation Techniques, Conflict Reduction and Prevention so that you can increase the peace in your home, the productivity of your ministry, and the profitability of your business.

* * * * *

Christian Anger Management

Christian Anger Management teaches Biblical anger management tips and self help strategies to help you manage anger instead of letting it manage you and destroy your testimony, life, family, and career.

* * * * *

Managing Stress For Teens

Managing Stress for Teens teaches teenagers Biblical principles, medical techniques, and life skills to manage 80 common teenage stressors.

It teaches them how to resist using alcohol, cigarettes, drugs, and how to overcome addiction. It edifies them to resist sexual temptation, fornication, pornography, homosexuality, and lesbianism. It also helps them cope with sickness, and disability.

Managing Stress for Teens also teaches teenagers how to manage emotions such as anger, anxiety, confusion, fear, guilt, loneliness, love, lust, low self confidence, and shyness. It guides them on how to deal with negative peer pressure. It also trains them to cope with family problems like abuse.

Managing Stress for Teens suggests constructive activities for teens who don't have money. It helps also helps them understand parental issues like pressure from parents and schools them on the best way to deal with bullying.

Managing Stress for Teens also clarifies issues on God, Jesus, The Holy Spirit, feeling they lack faith, and living right. It coaches them on how to deal with fashion trends, crime, corruption, and cultural practices. It also helps them understand puberty, their body shape, self image, gender realization and the effects of negative thoughts and words as well as helping them answer the questions "Who am I?" and "Why am I here?"

* * * * *

Dark Skin Dermatology Color Atlas

Dark Skin Dermatology Color Atlas is filled with clear explanations and color photos of skin, hair, and nail diseases affecting people with skin of color or Fitzpatrick skin types IV, V, and VI.

Topics covered include Acne Vulgaris, Alopecia Areata, Anal Warts, Angioedema, Aphthous Ulcers, Atopic Dermatitis, Blastomycosis, Blister Beetle Dermatitis or Nairobi Fly Dermatitis, Cellulitis, Chronic Ulcers, Confetti Hypopigmentation, Cutaneous T Cell Lymphoma, Cutaneous Tuberculosis, Dermatitis Artefacta, Erythema Nodosum, Exfoliative Erythroderma, Gianotti Crosti Syndrome, Hand Dermatitis , Hemangioma, Herpes Zoster, Ichthyosis, Ingrown Toenails, Irritant Contact Dermatitis, Kaposi Sarcoma, Keloids, Keratoderma Blenorrhagica, Klippel Trenaunay Weber Syndrome, Leishmaniasis, Leprosy, Leukonychia, Lichen Nitidus, Lichen Planus, Lichenoid Drug Eruption, Linear Epidermal Nevus, Linear IgA Dermatosis (LAD), Lipodermatosclerosis, Lymphangioma Circumscriptum, Miliaria, Molluscum Contagiosum, Neurofibromatosis, Nickel Dermatitis, Onychomadesis, Onychomycosis, Palmoplantar Eccrine Hidradenitis, Papular Pruritic Eruption (PPE), Paronychia, Pellagra, Pemphigus Foliaceous, Pemphigus Vulgaris, Piebaldism, Pityriasis Rosea, Pityriasis Rubra Pilaris, Plantar Hyperkeratosis, Plantar Warts, Poikiloderma, Postinflammatory Hyperpigmentation and Hypopigmentation, Post Topical Steroids Hypopigmentation, Psoriasis, Pyogenic Granuloma or Lobular Capillary Hemangioma, Scabies, Seborrheic Dermatitis, Steven Johnson Syndrome (SJS) and Toxic Epidermal Necrolysis (TEN), Sunburn, Systemic Sclerosis, Tinea Capitis, Tinea Pedis, Tinea Versicolor, Traction Alopecia, Urticaria, Vasculitis, Vitiligo, and Xanthelasma.

* * * * *

www.ingramcontent.com/pod-product-compliance
Lightning Source LLC
Chambersburg PA
CBHW070124010626
45794CB00012B/1280